I. Introduction

In U.S. v. Mercy, a U.S. District Court found that a merger between the only two

hospitals serving Dubuque, Iowa would not reduce competition because the merged hospital

would compete with hospitals 70-100 miles distant.[1] Similarly, in F.T.C. v Tenet, a U.S. Circuit

Court found that a merger between the only two hospitals in Poplar Bluff, Missouri would not

reduce competition because the merged hospital would continue to face competition from

hospitals 40-60 miles distant.[2] In reaching this conclusion, this court discounted statements by

insurers and large employers that their participants would be unlikely to use hospitals outside the

Poplar Bluff region in the event of a price increase at the merged hospital. Finally, in State of

California v. Sutter Health System, a U.S. District Court found that a merger of the two premier

hospitals in the Oakland/Berkeley area would not substantially lessen competition because the

merging hospitals would continue to face competition from hospitals 15-30 miles distant.[3]

Following the U.S. Department of Justice and Federal Trade Commission Merger

Guidelines, the courts in all three of these cases sought to define the geographic market as the

smallest area in which a "hypothetical monopolist" of all hospital services could profitably

increase price by a small but significant amount. Using this methodology, the courts then found

very broad geographic markets based on the following combination of economic theory, facts,

and assumptions: In each of these cases, both the plaintiffs and the defendants agreed that

hospitals have relatively high fixed costs and relatively low variable costs and therefore earn high

---

[1] United States v. Mercy Health Servs., 902 F.Supp. 968 (N.D. Iowa 1995) vacated as moot 107 F.3d 632 (8th Cir. 1997).

[2] F.T.C. v. Tenet Healthcare Corp., 186 F.3d 1045 (8th Cir. 1999).

[3] State of California v. Sutter Health System, et al, No. C99-03803 MMC, at 24 (N.D. Cal. 2000)

profits on the last patients that they serve. Given that hospitals earn high profits on the last patients that they serve, economic theory indicates that a small price increase (e.g., 5 percent) would be unprofitable if even a relatively small percentage (e.g., 8 percent) of patients switched to more distant hospitals.[4] In each of these cases, many of the patients who used the merging hospitals lived in contestable zip codes, which are zip codes where a large percentage of patients already use other hospitals. The defendants in these cases argued that many of the patients that use a merging hospital and live in contestable zip codes would switch to other hospitals if the merging hospitals increased price. The defendants then argued that this amount of switching would make any price increase unprofitable. The courts in each of these cases accepted this argument by the defendants.

This paper argues that the courts in these cases erred in accepting the defendants' argument that switching by patients living in contestable zip codes would make a price increase at the merging hospitals unprofitable. Specifically, this paper examines the behavior of patients following a merger similar to those analyzed by these courts and finds that a large price increase prompted little switching by those patients that used the merging hospitals and lived in contestable zip codes. Section II of this paper describes 259-bed Dominican Santa Cruz Hospital's (Dominican) 1990 acquisition of 180-bed Community Hospital (Community), the only other general acute-care hospital serving Santa Cruz, California. Section III discusses the data, variables, and model that are used to study the effects of this acquisition.

_____

[4] If a hospital has a profit margin of 60 percent on the last patients that it treats, then a 5 percent price increase would be unprofitable if this hospital lost about 8 percent of its patients. See Langenfeld, J., and W. Li, Critical Loss Analysis in Evaluating Mergers, Antitrust Bulletin, forthcoming, for a discussion of the amount of switching that makes various price increases unprofitable.

Section IV finds that the price for hospital care in Santa Cruz increased following Dominican's acquisition of Community by at least 5 percent relative to the price at neighboring hospitals. While this price increase suggests that demand for hospital care in Santa Cruz was not sufficiently elastic to make the price increase unprofitable, by itself, this price increase does not indicate whether patients in contestable zip codes change hospitals in response to relative price changes. To answer this question, Section V analyzes changes in patient flow in several clusters of contestable zip codes after the price increase. Section V finds that the relative price increase for hospital care in Santa Cruz led to very little switching to other hospitals even in these contestable areas. Section VI concludes.

II. Dominican Santa Cruz Hospital's acquisition of Community Hospital

The city of Santa Cruz is located on the coast of California approximately 70 miles south of San Francisco and approximately 30 miles southwest of San Jose. Prior to 1990, two general acute care hospitals, 259-bed Dominican and 180-bed Community had served Santa Cruz. Watsonville Community Hospital (Watsonville), a 112-bed general acute-care hospital, is located in Watsonville which is approximately 14 miles east of Santa Cruz. Several large general acute care hospitals are located about 30 miles northeast of Santa Cruz in the San Jose metropolitan area.

Dominican acquired Community in March 1990 and converted it to a nursing home/rehabilitation facility five months later. The Federal Trade Commission (FTC) began an investigation of this acquisition shortly after it occurred. As a result of this investigation, the

4

FTC concluded that the acquisition likely reduced competition for inpatient acute care services.[5] However, the FTC did not attempt to force Dominican to divest Community for two reasons. First, the FTC concluded that converting Community back to a full-service hospital would be very costly with no guarantee of success. Second, the FTC believed that the proposed entry of a small hospital might pose a competitive check on Dominican. The FTC, however, did obtain a consent decree which required that Dominican obtain the FTC's approval before acquiring any other hospitals in Santa Cruz County. In March 1996, 30-bed Sutter Maternity and Surgery Center opened in Santa Cruz.

III. Data, Variable Descriptions, and Model

This study uses two data sets from the California Office of Statewide Health Planning and Development (OSHPD) to analyze the effect of Dominican's acquisition of Community on hospital prices and then the effect of this price change on patient flow. The first data set, which contains financial data for each hospital in California, is used to compute a measure of the price paid by privately-insured patients at various hospitals.[6] Specifically, a hospital's net revenue for privately-insured patients is computed by multiplying the total net revenues from these patients by the ratio of gross inpatient revenue from these patients to the gross total (inpatient and

---

[5] See Statement of Chairman Janet D. Steiger in Support of Final Issuance of Consent Order in the Matter of Dominican Santa Cruz, et al. Federal Trade Commission Decisions, Volume 118, pp 382-394.

[6] Presumably, post-merger anticompetitive behavior will most likely take the form of a price increase directed at privately-insured patients. For this reason, this study focuses on "privately-insured" patients, those patients who are not covered by either Medicare or Medicaid. The vast majority of these patients have some form of private insurance although some of these patients are indigent.

outpatient) revenue from these patients. Dividing this estimate by the privately-insured

discharges yields the average net revenue for a privately-insured inpatient acute-care discharge.[7]

OSHPD also compiles annual data for each inpatient discharge for each hospital in

California. This data includes information on a patient's diagnosis (DRG). Each year, the

Health Care Financing Administration (HCFA) computes DRG weights based on their estimate

of the resources needed to treat a particular DRG. Assigning the appropriate DRG weight to

each discharge and then taking the average of these weights across all of a hospital's privately-

insured discharges yields a case mix index that measures the relative complexity of care provided

by a hospital to its privately-insured patients.

Dividing each hospital's average net revenue for a privately-insured inpatient acute-care

discharge by its case mix index for privately-insured patients yields the measure of price used in

this study. The measures of relative price are then the price of hospital care at Dominican

divided by the price of hospital care at neighboring hospitals. [8]

OSHPD's patient discharge data set also provides information on a patient's zip code,

which can be used to compute market share. Specifically, for several zip code clusters, market

share is computed as the sum of Dominican's and Community's privately-insured acute-care

---

[7] A hospital's price can be measured as price per discharge or price per day. This paper uses price per discharge for the following reason. If competition among hospitals leads to shorter stays for a discharge, then a decrease in competition may result in an increase in the number of patient days required to treat a discharge. In this case, measuring price as price per day may understate the quality-adjusted price increase following this acquisition.

[8] The relative changes in price can be computed using Dominican's pre-acquisition prices or a weighted average of Dominican's and Community's pre-acquisition prices. This paper uses Dominican's pre-acquisition prices since using Dominican's prices throughout avoids any measurement error that might be caused by different accounting practices or levels of care at the two hospitals.

discharges divided by the total number of privately-insured acute-care discharges. These acute-care discharges exclude diagnoses for the following: psychiatric care, drug and alcohol rehabilitation, physical rehabilitation, and normal delivery (because the newborn is already counted).

The data on price and market share is limited to the time period beginning in 1986 and ending in 1996. The data set does not go back prior to 1986 because OSHPD did not collect sufficient data at that time. The data set does not extend past 1996 because entry by Sutter Maternity and Surgery Center created market conditions different than both those in the 1986-1989 period and those in the 1990-1996 period. This paper treats each of the eleven years between 1986 and 1996 as a separate observation for the following reason.[9] Patient flow is largely determined by contracts between providers and insurers and contracts between insurers and employers (and their employees). Since these contracts tend to be negotiated annually, this study treats each year as an observation.

For both the observations of relative price and the observations of market share, the four pre-merger observations can be viewed as an independent random sample from a continuous distribution and the seven post-merger observations can be viewed as an independent random sample potentially from a different continuous distribution. Given this, we want to test the extent to which these underlying distributions have different means. Unfortunately, because the two samples are very small, we cannot use the Central Limit Theorem to infer that the sample means are normally distributed. As a result, to obtain a test statistic, we are forced to make some assumption about the underlying pre-merger and post-merger distributions.

_____

[9] The results change little if 1996, the year of Sutter's entry, is dropped from the sample.

If we assume that the underlying distributions have the same shape and spread, then the Wilcoxon Rank Sum Test can determine the extent to which the means of the underlying distributions differ.[10] To do this, the Wilcoxon Rank-Sum Test begins by combining the two samples. If one sample is drawn from a distribution with a much higher mean than the distribution generating the second sample, then the observations from the first sample would be higher than the observations from the second sample. However, if the two samples are drawn from the same distribution, the observations from the two samples would be intermingled.

The Wilcoxon Rank-Sum Test quantifies the extent to which the two samples are intermingled. Specifically, the Wilcoxon Rank-Sum Test assigns each observation in the combined sample a rank (e.g., 1, 3). The Wilcoxon Rank-Sum Test then sums the ranks of the smaller sample. If the sum of these ranks falls above or below a critical level, which varies depending on the size of the samples and the chosen level of statistical significance, the Wilcoxon Rank-Sum Test rejects at the chosen level of statistical significance the null hypothesis that the two samples have the same mean. For a sample of four pre-merger observations and a sample of seven post-merger observations, the critical level to reject a null hypothesis at the 0.05 level is below 16 or above 32.

The null hypothesis that the mean of one distribution exceeds the mean of another sample by a given amount, say 5 percent, can be analyzed by reducing the first sample by 5 percent, ranking the new values, and then testing to see whether the first sample overwhelmingly has the

_____

[10] The Wilcoxon Rank-Sum Test (Mann-Whitney test) is a non-parametric test that can be used to determine if two small samples are drawn from different distributions. This test assumes that the two distributions have exactly the same shape and spread but does not assume that the two distributions are normally distributed. For a more detailed description of the Wilcoxon Rank-Sum Test see Devore, Jay, 1982, Probability & Statistics for Engineering and the Sciences, Brooks/Cole Publishing Company, Monterey, CA.

high ranks. In analyzing various pairs of samples, this study seeks null hypotheses about changes in price or changes in market share that will be rejected at level 0.05. As a consequence, the null hypotheses used in this study (i.e., changes in price, changes in market share) will vary depending on the particular samples examined.

The Wilcoxon Rank Sum Test only assumes that the two underlying distributions have the same shape and spread. If we make the stronger assumption that the two underlying distributions are normal distributions with the same variance, then we can use a t-test to determine whether the two distributions have the same mean. For many of the null hypotheses tested with the Wilcoxon Rank Sum Test, this paper also tests the null hypothesis with a t-test.

IV. Evidence of a Post-Merger Price Increase

Several types of evidence indicate that prices at Dominican increased relative to prices at nearby hospitals following the acquisition. Table 1 shows the price at Dominican divided by the price at Good Samaritan Hospital in San Jose. This ratio is important because Good Samaritan Hospital drew more patients from the zip codes just east of Santa Cruz than any hospital except Dominican or Community. The data in Table 1 show that prices at Dominican rose relative to the prices at Good Samaritan Hospital after the acquisition. Given these data, the Wilcoxon Rank Sum Test enables us to test whether the seven annual post-merger price ratios were 5 percent higher than the four annual pre-merger price ratios. Row 1 lists the Dominican/Good Samaritan price ratios. Row 2 inflates the pre-merger price ratios by 5 percent, and Row 3 ranks these eleven ratios. The sum of the pre-merger ranks, 14, enables us to reject at level 0.05 the null hypothesis that the post-merger price ratios were less than 5 percent higher than the pre-merger price ratios. The results of a t-test are presented below Table 1. Given these results, the

9

t-test rejects at level 0.03 the null hypothesis that the post-merger prices were less than 5 percent higher than the pre-merger prices. These results suggest that prices at Dominican increased by at least 5 percent relative to prices at Good Samaritan.

Table 1
Relative increases in Dominican's price

	1986	1987	1988	1989	1990	1991	1992	1993	1994	1995	1996
Dominican's price / Good Samaritan's price	0.839	0.860	0.800	0.807	1.025	1.006	1.040	0.925	0.889	0.843	0.943
pre-merger ratio increased by 5 %	0.881	0.903	0.840	0.847	1.025	1.006	1.040	0.925	0.889	0.843	0.943
ranks	4	6	1	3	10	9	11	7	5	2	8

pre-merger (row 2) mean	0.868	t-statistic	2.17
post-merger mean	0.953	p-value	0.03
standard error	0.039		

Table 2 shows the price at Dominican divided by the price at Watsonville. This ratio is important because Watsonville is Dominican's primary competitor in those zip codes southeast of Santa Cruz. The data in Table 2 show that prices at Dominican rose relative to the prices at Watsonville after the acquisition. Rows 1,2, and 3, present the Wilcoxon Rank-Sum analysis for the Dominican/Watsonville price ratios. Once again, the sum of the pre-merger ranks, 15, enables us to reject at level 0.05 the null hypothesis that the post-merger price ratios were less than 5 percent higher than the pre-merger price ratios.[11] A t-test, however, fails to reject at level

---

[11]   If the relative prices are calculated by patient day rather than by patient discharge, post-acquisition relative prices are still higher than pre-acquisition relative prices, however, the level of statistical significance falls. If the pre-merger relative prices are calculated for a combined Dominican and Community rather than for just Dominican, the post-acquisition relative prices are still higher than the pre-acquisition relative prices, however, the level of

10

0.05 the null hypothesis that the post-merger prices were less than 5 percent higher than the pre-merger prices, but does reject this null hypothesis at level 0.06. On balance, these results suggest that prices at Dominican increased by at least 5 percent relative to prices at Watsonville.

Table 2
Relative increases in Dominican's price

	1986	1987	1988	1989	1990	1991	1992	1993	1994	1995	1996
Dominican's price / Watsonville's price	0.812	0.910	1.058	1.043	1.233	0.801	1.142	1.108	1.382	1.538	1.448
pre-merger ratio increased by 5%	0.853	0.956	1.111	1.095	1.233	0.801	1.142	1.108	1.382	1.538	1.448
ranks	2	3	6	4	8	1	7	5	9	11	10

pre-merger (row 2) mean	1.004	t-statistic	1.723
post-merger mean	1.235	p-value	0.06
standard error	0.135		

The results in Tables 1 and 2 are consistent with results found by Vita and Sacher (2000).[12] For the time period 1986-1996, they compare prices at Dominican with the prices at various peer hospitals throughout California. After adjusting for changes in quality, they find that the case-mix adjusted price of an inpatient admission at Dominican relative to the case-mix adjusted price of an inpatient admission at these peer hospitals increased by 23 percent after the acquisition. They also find that the case-mix adjusted price of an inpatient admission at Watsonville relative to the price at these peer hospitals increased by 17 percent after the

statistical significance falls.

[12] Vita, Michael, and Seth Sacher, 2001, "The competitive effects of not-for-profit hospital mergers: A case study," Journal of Industrial Economics, forthcoming.

acquisition. Given this, their results suggest that Dominican's prices increased by about 5-6 percent relative to Watsonville's prices.

Finally, as noted above, 30-bed Sutter Maternity and Surgery Center opened in Santa Cruz several years after Dominican acquired Community. Entry by a hospital is profitable only where the entrant can obtain enough sales to operate at some minimum viable scale. Thus, the most likely targets for new entry are areas with rapid population growth and areas where the incumbent hospital is currently setting a high price and restricting output. During the early 1990s, very few hospitals entered de novo in California.[13] Of those that did, many entered rapidly growing suburbs of large cities (e.g., San Ramon, Gilroy). In contrast, the population in Santa Cruz grew at a significantly slower rate than the population of the state of California. Given this, Sutter's entry seems to suggest that the incumbent producer, Dominican, was setting high prices and restricting output.

V. Post-merger changes in patient flow

The previous section found that hospital prices in Santa Cruz increased relative to prices at neighboring hospitals following Dominican's acquisition of Community. This section examines how patients responded to this price increase. The zip codes listed in Table 3 contributed over 95 percent of the patients at the two Santa Cruz hospitals for the years 1986 to 1989. Column 1 lists these zip codes, and column 2 lists the corresponding city. Column 3 lists the total number of patients from each zip code who used one of the Santa Cruz hospitals. Column 4 lists the percentage of patients from each zip code who obtained care at the Santa

---

[13] See Simpson, John, 1995, "A note on entry by small hospitals," Journal of Health Economics, 14, 107-113.

Table 3
Geographic Areas Served by Santa Cruz Hospitals (SC)

zipcode	city	patients using SC	percent using SC	percent of SC patients	area
95060	Santa Cruz	5897	81.5	21.0	1 Santa Cruz area
95062	Santa Cruz	4681	83.8	16.6	1 Santa Cruz area
95065	Santa Cruz	1024	76.2	3.6	1 Santa Cruz area
95064	Santa Cruz	154	82.3	0.5	1 Santa Cruz area
95061	Santa Cruz	139	79.4	0.5	1 Santa Cruz area
95063	Santa Cruz	91	75.2	0.3	1 Santa Cruz area
95073	Soquel	1442	77.8	5.1	1 Santa Cruz area
95010	Capitola	1339	78.0	4.8	1 Santa Cruz area
95017	Davenport	102	81.6	0.4	1 Santa Cruz area
95066	Scotts Valley	1662	78.5	5.9	2 Ben Lomond area
95018	Felton	1193	75.4	4.2	2 Ben Lomond area
95006	Ben Lomond	1015	56.5	3.6	2 Ben Lomond area
95005	Boulder Creek	965	71.0	3.4	2 Ben Lomond area
95041	Mount Hermon	137	65.0	0.5	2 Ben Lomond area
95007	Brookdale	123	72.9	0.4	2 Ben Lomond area
95003	Aptos	2829	70.2	10.1	3 Aptos
95001	Aptos	83	58.8	0.3	3 Aptos
95076	Watsonville	3092	21.3	11.0	4 Watsonville area
95019	Freedom	207	19.8	0.7	4 Watsonville area
95004	Aromas	101	17.4	0.4	4 Watsonville area
95030	Los Gatos	180	2.4	0.6	5 Outlying area
95012	Castroville	65	3.2	0.2	5 Outlying area
95023	Hollister	57	0.9	0.2	5 Outlying area
93907	Salinas	51	1.1	0.2	5 Outlying area
94060	Pescadero	43	11.1	0.2	5 Outlying area
95020	Gilroy	42	0.4	0.1	5 Outlying area
93906	Salinas	38	0.4	0.1	5 Outlying area
95008	Campbell	35	0.4	0.1	5 Outlying area
93901	Salinas	30	1.0	0.1	5 Outlying area

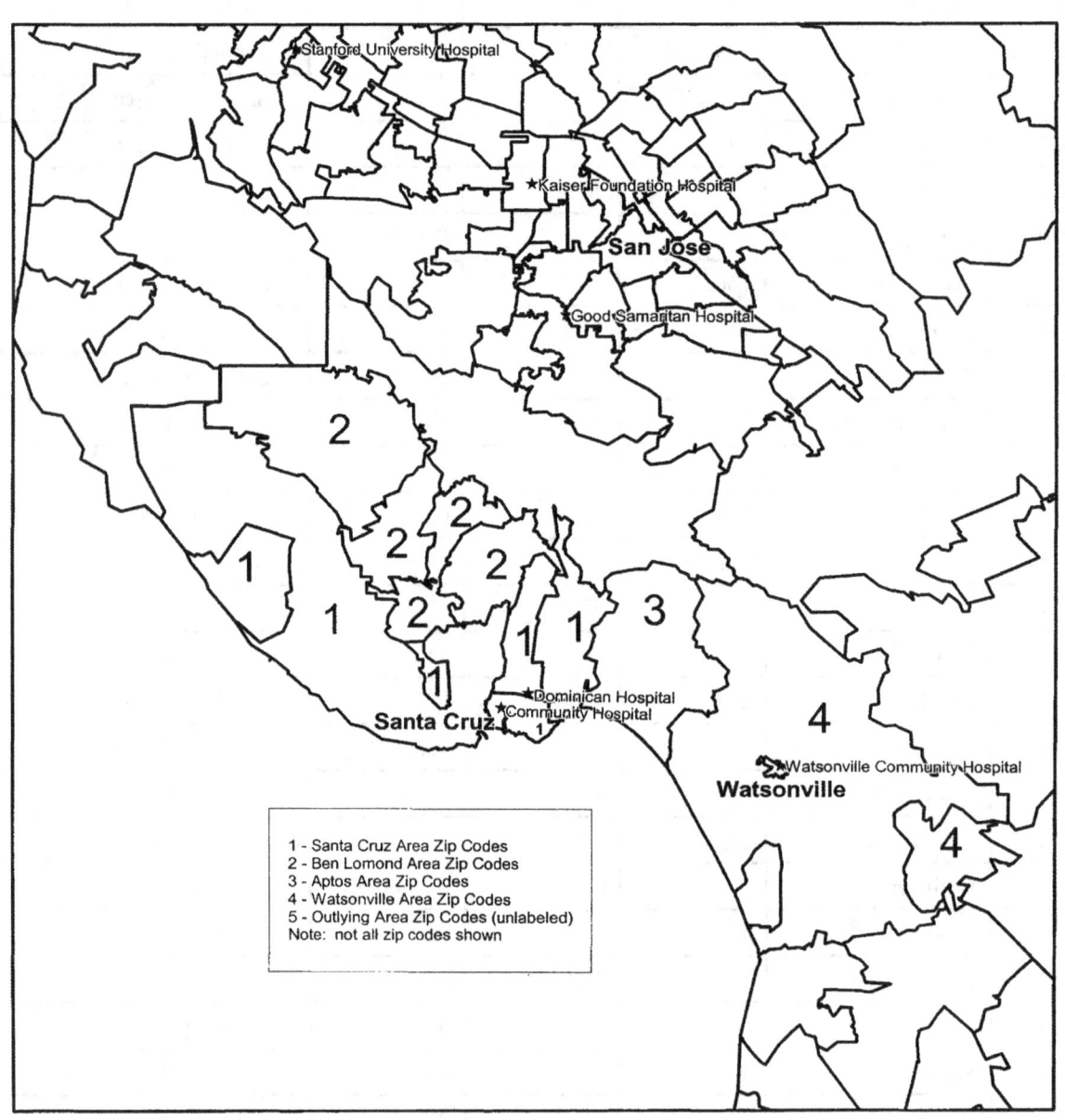

1 inch=7.3 miles

Cruz hospitals. Column 5 lists the percentage of patient discharges at the Santa Cruz hospitals accounted for by each zip code. Based on the location of these zip codes and the information in columns 4 and 5, we can divide the service area of the Santa Cruz hospitals into five areas, the Santa Cruz area, the Brookdale area, Aptos, the Watsonville area, and outlying areas. These areas are listed in column 6 of Table 3 and are shown in the map on the following page. In all of these areas except the Santa Cruz area, more than 20 percent of the patients sought care at hospitals other than the Santa Cruz hospitals.

The Santa Cruz area is comprised of the first nine zip codes listed in Table 3. The two Santa Cruz hospitals received about 53 percent of their admissions from this area, and about 80 percent of the patients living in this area used one of the two Santa Cruz hospitals. About 11 percent of the patients living in this area used hospitals in Santa Clara County, which includes the city of San Jose. Stanford University Hospital received the largest number of these patients (3.1 percent), and Good Samaritan Hospital received the second largest number of these patients (2 percent). Based on their geographic location, we would expect that patients living in these zip codes would be the patients least likely to switch away from the Santa Cruz hospitals.

Row 1 of Table 4 shows the combined market share of Dominican and Community from 1986 to 1996. Given these data, the Wilcoxon Rank Sum Test enables us to test whether the seven annual post-merger market share observations were smaller than the four annual pre-merger market share observations. Row 2 ranks the market share observations. The sum of the ranks of the pre-merger market shares, 37, enables us to reject at level 0.02 the null hypothesis that the post-merger market shares equal or exceed the pre-merger market shares. This suggests that Dominican's post-merger price increase led to a decline in its market share in the Santa Cruz area.

15

Table 4
Market Share Changes - Santa Cruz Area

	1986	1987	1988	1989	1990	1991	1992	1993	1994	1995	1996
pre-merger shares (unadjusted)	82.1	80.4	79.8	82.1	80.2	79.4	78.2	78.8	78.5	79.7	74.5
rank	11	9	7	10	8	5	2	4	3	6	1
pre-merger shares reduced by 5 percent	78.0	76.4	75.8	78.0	80.2	79.4	78.2	78.8	78.5	79.7	74.5
rank	5	3	2	4	11	9	6	8	7	10	1

pre-merger (row 3) mean   77.05   t-statistic   1.36
post-merger mean   78.47   p-value   0.10
standard error   1.05

The Wilcoxon Rank Sum Test also enables us to test whether the post-merger market share is 5 percent below the pre-merger market share. To do this, the pre-merger market shares are reduced by 5 percent in row 3, and the new market shares are ranked in Row 4. The sum of the ranks of the adjusted pre-merger market shares, 14, enables us to reject at level 0.05 the null hypothesis that market share fell by more than 5 percent post-merger. A t-test rejects at level 0.10 the null hypothesis that market share fell by more than 5 percent post-merger. Thus, while the post-merger price increase at Dominican likely led to a decline in market share in the Santa Cruz area, the decline was likely less than 5 percent.

The Ben Lomond area, the tenth through fifteenth zip codes listed in Table 3, is comprised of the small cities lying to the north and northwest of Santa Cruz. The location of this area is such that travel to San Jose takes about twice as long as travel into Santa Cruz. The two Santa Cruz hospitals received about 18 percent of their admissions from this area, and 66.4 percent of the patients in this area used the Santa Cruz hospitals. About 26 percent of the patients living in this area used hospitals in Santa Clara County. Good Samaritan Hospital received the largest share of these patients (6.4 percent) and Kaiser Hospital - Santa Clara received the second largest share of these patients (5.5 percent).

Row 1 of Table 5 shows the market shares of Dominican and Community in the Ben Lomond area. Row 2 shows the ranks for the market shares of Dominican and Community. The sum of the ranks of the pre-merger market shares, 31, does not enable us to reject at level 0.05 the null hypothesis that the post-merger market shares equal or exceed the pre-merger market shares. Row 4 shows the ranks when the pre-merger market shares have been reduced by 6 percent.[14] The sum of the ranks of these adjusted pre-merger market shares, 13, enables us to reject at level 0.02 the null hypothesis that market share fell by more than 5 percent post-merger. A t-test also rejects this null hypothesis at level 0.02. This suggests that the post-merger price increase at Dominican led to very little switching in the Ben Lomond area.

---

[14] The pre-merger market shares are reduced by 6 percent rather than 5 percent so that the null hypothesis can be rejected at level 0.05 using the Wilcoxon Rank Sum Test.

Table 5
Market Share Changes - Ben Lomond Area

	1986	1987	1988	1989	1990	1991	1992	1993	1994	1995	1996
pre-merger shares (unadjusted)	70.5	67.0	65.5	68.4	64.7	67.1	65.4	64.6	67.5	66.6	67.3
rank	11	6	4	10	2	7	3	1	9	5	8
pre-merger shares reduced by 6 percent	66.3	63.0	61.6	64.3	64.7	67.1	65.4	64.6	67.5	66.6	67.3
rank	7	2	1	3	5	9	6	4	11	8	10

pre-merger (row 3) mean	63.78	t-statistic	2.48
post-merger mean	66.17	p-value	0.02
standard error	0.96		

The city of Aptos is located about five miles east of Santa Cruz and ten miles west of Watsonville. The two zip codes in Aptos accounted for 10 percent of the admissions at the Santa Cruz hospitals, and about 68 percent of patients in Aptos used Santa Cruz hospitals. Of the remaining patients, 8 percent used Watsonville Community Hospital, and 14 percent used hospitals in Santa Clara County. Row 2 of Table 6 shows the ranks for the market shares of Dominican and Community. As with the Ben Lomond area, the sum of the ranks of the pre-merger market shares, 31, does not enable us to reject at level 0.05 the null hypothesis that the post-merger market shares equal or exceed the pre-merger market shares. Row 3 reduces the pre-merger market shares by 5 percent. The sum of the ranks of these adjusted pre-merger market shares, 15, enables us to reject at level 0.05 the null hypothesis that the post-merger market shares fell by more than 5 percent. A t-test enables us to reject this null hypothesis at level 0.04. This suggests that the post-merger price increase at Dominican led to very little switching in the Aptos area.

Table 6
Market Share Changes - Aptos Area

	1986	1987	1988	1989	1990	1991	1992	1993	1994	1995	1996
pre-merger shares (unadjusted)	70.3	70.6	69.6	69.4	66.3	69.7	71.5	66.9	66.5	70.7	68.5
rank	8	9	6	5	1	7	11	3	2	10	4
pre-merger shares reduced by 5 percent	66.8	67.1	66.1	65.9	66.3	69.7	71.5	66.9	66.5	70.7	68.5
rank	5	7	2	1	3	9	11	6	4	10	8

pre-merger (row 3) mean	66.48	t-statistic	1.93
post-merger mean	68.59	p-value	0.04
standard error	1.10		

19

The Watsonville area includes Watsonville, Freedom, and Aromas. Patients from this area comprised 12 percent of the patients at Santa Cruz hospitals, and 21.1 percent of the patients in this area used Santa Cruz hospitals. About 59 percent of the patients in this area used Watsonville Community Hospital. Row 1 of Table 7 shows the market shares of Dominican and Santa Cruz in the Watsonville area, and Row 2 shows the ranks of these market shares. As with the Ben Lomond area and the Aptos area, the sum of the ranks of the pre-merger market shares, 19, does not enable us to reject at level 0.05 the null hypothesis that the post-merger market shares equal or exceed the pre-merger market shares. Row 3 reduces the pre-merger market shares by 5 percent. The sum of the ranks of these adjusted pre-merger market shares, 13, enables us to reject at level 0.02 the null hypothesis that post-merger market shares fell by more than 5 percent. A t-test also enables us to reject at level 0.01 this null hypothesis. This suggests that the post-merger price increase at Dominican led to very little switching in the Watsonville area.

Table 7
Market Share Changes - Watsonville Area

	1986	1987	1988	1989	1990	1991	1992	1993	1994	1995	1996
pre-merger shares (unadjusted)	19.7	20.8	21.9	21.6	21.5	20.5	22.2	21.7	20.8	23.8	24.3
rank	1	4	8	6	5	2	9	7	3	10	11
pre-merger shares reduced by 5 percent	18.7	19.8	20.8	20.5	21.5	20.5	22.2	21.7	20.8	23.8	24.3
rank	1	2	6	4	7	3	9	8	5	10	11

pre-merger (row 3) mean	19.95		t-statistic	2.66
post-merger mean	22.11		p-value	0.01
standard error	0.81			

Finally, about 8 percent of the patients at the Santa Cruz hospitals came from more distant areas (e.g., Los Gatos, Salinas, Hollister). On average, the Santa Cruz hospitals obtained a very small share of the patients from these zip codes (e.g 1 percent). Table 7 shows whether the post-merger price increase at Domincan led to switching in the nine outlying zip codes that sent the most patients to Dominican. The sum of the ranks of the pre-merger market shares, 30, does not allow us to reject at level 0.05 the null hypothesis that the post-merger market shares equal or exceed the pre-merger market shares. Row 3 of Table 7 reduces the pre-merger market shares by 25 percent. The sum of the ranks of these adjusted pre-merger market shares, 15, enables us to reject at level 0.05 the null hypothesis that post-merger market shares fell by more than 25 percent. A t-test enables us to reject at level 0.01 this null hypothesis. This suggests that Dominican's post-merger increase in price led to at most a 25 percent decline in its market share in the outlying areas that provided about 7 percent of its patient base.

Table 8
Market Share Changes - Outlying Zip Codes

	1986	1987	1988	1989	1990	1991	1992	1993	1994	1995	1996
pre-merger shares (unadjusted)	0.82	1.09	1.14	1.23	0.96	0.91	0.90	0.94	0.91	1.10	0.82
rank	1	8	10	11	7	4	3	6	5	9	2
pre-merger shares reduced by 25 percent	0.62	0.81	0.85	0.92	0.96	0.91	0.90	0.94	0.91	1.10	0.82
rank	1	2	4	8	10	6	5	9	7	11	3

pre-merger (row 3) mean   0.76   t-statistic   2.75

post-merger mean   0.93   p-value   0.01

standard error   0.063

VI. Conclusion

In three recent hospital merger cases, the courts concluded that the merged hospital would be unable to increase price profitably because of competition from distant hospitals. In reaching this conclusion the courts found the following: hospitals earn high margins on the last patients that they serve; given these high margins, a small price increase would be unprofitable if even a relatively small percentage of patients switched to other hospitals; many of the merging hospitals' patients live in zip codes where a large percentage of patients already use other hospitals; a price increase at the merging hospitals would prompt a large number of these patients to switch to other hospitals; and this amount of switching would make the price increase unprofitable.

This paper examines Dominican's 1990 acquisition of Community, which was similar to the mergers described above, and finds that a price increase at the merged hospital led to very little switching to neighboring hospitals. In three areas, accounting for 75 percent of the admissions at the Santa Cruz hospitals, the price increase led to less than a 5 percent decline in market share. Two of these areas, Aptos and the Watsonville area, would have been viewed by the courts as "contestable." In one other area, the Ben Lomond area, which the courts also would have labeled as "contestable," the price increase led to less than a 6 percent decline in market share. In the fifth area, accounting for only 7 percent of the admissions at the Santa Cruz hospitals, the price increase led to at most a 25 percent decline in market share.

The results found here presumably would apply to at least some other cases involving the merger of the only two hospitals serving an isolated city. To show this, Table 9 compares certain key facts for the hospital merger in Santa Cruz with the facts for the hospital mergers in Poplar Bluff and Dubuque. Row 1 looks at the distance separating the merging hospitals from the next best alterative, and row 2 lists the travel time required to cover this distance. Since patients living in contestable zip codes presumably will need to travel longer distances as the distance between the merging hospitals and the next best alternatives increase, this measure of travel should represent a crude measure of the travel time that a patient living in a contestable zip code must bear to get to the more distant hospital. Using this measure, the travel times for patients living in contestable zip codes would have been about 3 times as long for the mergers in Poplar Bluff and Dubuque as for the merger in Santa Cruz.

Row 3 looks at the geographic location of the merging hospitals' patients relative to the merging hospital and the next best alternatives. Of the three mergers shown, the relative distance to the next best hospital appears to be greatest for patients at the Dubuque hospital. Row 4 looks at the percentage of the merging hospitals' patients that come from contestable zip codes, which are defined here as zip codes where 20 percent of the patients already choose other hospitals. Of the three mergers shown, the Santa Cruz hospitals have the highest percentage of patients living in contestable zip codes.

Row 5 looks at the per capita income in the counties in which the three mergers occurred. Per capita income represents a crude measure of the cost to a patient of traveling. Using this measure, Santa Cruz patients have a cost of traveling that is about 30 percent higher than that of Dubuque patients and about 40 percent higher than that of Poplar Bluff patients. Since the cost to a patient of switching to an alternative hospital is the product of the travel time and the cost of travel, the cost of switching is probably no higher for the Santa Cruz patients than for the Poplar Bluff patients or Dubuque patients.

Row 6 looks at managed care penetration in the three areas. In contrast to traditional fee-for-service plans, managed care plans create significant incentives for patients to use lower cost health providers. Thus, patients should be more willing to travel in areas where managed care penetration is high than in areas where managed care penetration is low. Given this, the figures in row 4 suggest that patients in Santa Cruz would be more willing than patients in Poplar Bluff or Dubuque to travel to avoid higher hospital prices.

Table 9 examines some of the key factors that would affect a patients's willingness to travel. Based on these factors, the patients at the Santa Cruz hospitals should be at least as willing as the patients at the Poplar Bluff hospitals and the Dubuque hospitals to travel to their next best alternative hospital. Thus, the finding that a 5 percent price increase at the Santa Cruz hospitals prompted only a very small percentage of patients at these hospitals to switch to more distant hospitals suggests that a 5 percent price increase at the Poplar Bluff hospitals and the Dubuque hospitals would likewise prompt only a very small percentage of the patients at these hospitals to switch to more distant hospitals. This, in turn, suggests that the courts in these two cases likely erred in concluding that competition from distant hospitals would prevent a price increase if the only two hospitals serving an isolated city merged.

Table 9

Comparison of Mergers in Santa Cruz, Dubuque, and Poplar Bluff

	Santa Cruz	Poplar Bluff	Dubuque
distance from merging hospitals to competing hospitals[4]	14 miles (Watsonville) 30 miles (San Jose)	40-60 miles	70-100 miles
travel time from merging hospitals to competing hospitals[4]	1/2 - 3/4 hours	1 1/2 - 2 hours	2 hours
location of merging hospitals' patients	43 percent from Santa Cruz, 77 percent within 10 miles.[1]	90 percent within 50 miles[2]	55 percent from Dubuque, 85 percent within 25 miles[2]
merging hospitals' patients in contestable zip codes	61.5 % live in zip codes where 1/5 go elsewhere.[1]	56.3 % live in zip codes where 1/5 go elsewhere.[3]	26.0 % live in zip codes where 1/5 go elsewhere.[3]
per-capita income[5]	$22,025	$12,795	$16,323
managed care penetration	over 80 percent of privately-insured patients in HMOs & PPOs[1]	few HMOs, many PPOs[2]	half of privately-insured patients in HMOs & PPOs[2]

[1] OSHPD discharge data set, [2] Respective court decisions, [3] Testimony of Barry Harris (defendant's expert), [4] Yahoo Maps,
[5] U.S. Bureau of the Census. County and City Data Book: 1994